Fatty Liver Diet

A Beginner's Step by Step Guide to Managing
Fatty Liver Disease

Includes Selected Recipes and a Meal Plan

Disclaimer

By reading this disclaimer, you are accepting the terms of the disclaimer in full. If you disagree with this disclaimer, please do not read the book. The content in this book is provided for informational and educational purposes only.

This book is not intended to be a substitute for the original work of this diet plan. At most, this book is intended to be beginner's supplement to the original work for this diet plan and never act as a direct substitute. This book, is an overview, review, and commentary of the facts of that diet plan.

All product names, diet plans, or names used in this book are for identification purposes only and are property of their respective owners. Use of these names does not imply endorsement. All other trademarks cited herein are property of their respective owners.
None of the information in this book should be accepted as independent medical or other professional advice.

Table of Contents

Introduction

I want to thank you and congratulate you for getting this guide.

Fatty liver is a condition that currently affects almost a third of the US population. This is mainly due to excessive alcohol consumption, unhealthy food choices, and sedentary lifestyles.

Left unchecked, fatty liver can cause damage to the liver and lead to serious medical conditions such as liver fibrosis or scarring, and cirrhosis, which can be fatal.

As of this writing, there are no FDA approved medications for the direct treatment of fatty liver. Fortunately, and if diagnosed early, this condition is easily reversible by making changes in the patient's diet and lifestyle.

That's where this guide can help. It's written for people who were diagnosed with fatty liver and are hoping to eat healthier.

The guide starts with important information on the disease and the symptoms that accompany it.

A chapter is devoted to listing the foods shown to help with the treatment and reversal of fatty liver according to studies. A diet and lifestyle change plan is also included in the guide to help the patient in the journey to living healthier.

Thanks again for getting this guide. I hope you enjoy it!

Chapter 1 – What is Fatty liver?

Also known as hepatic steatosis, fatty liver happens when there is a buildup of fat in the liver. Although it is normal to have a small amount of fat in the liver, too much of it can cause a serious health problem.

The liver is the human body's second-largest organ. Its basic function is to assist in the processing of nutrients from food and drinks and also filtering out harmful substances from the blood.

Too much fat in the liver can cause it to become inflamed. This can damage the liver and eventually cause irreversible damage or scarring and in severe cases, death.

If a person who drinks too much alcohol develops fatty liver, the condition is called alcoholic fatty liver or AFLD.

If a person who doesn't drink alcohol is diagnosed with the disease, it's called non-alcoholic fatty liver or NAFLD.

Currently, 25 to 30% of people in Europe and the United States are suffering from NAFLD according to a report released by researchers from the World Journal of Gastroenterology.

What are the Symptoms?

In most cases, fatty liver is asymptomatic which means there are no noticeable symptoms. Patients may initially experience general exhaustion or feel pain and discomfort in the upper right side of the abdomen.

When fatty liver is left unchecked, a person suffering from it can develop complications, one of which is liver scarring. This condition is called fibrosis and if it gets worse, it can lead to liver cirrhosis, a potentially deadly medical condition.

Some symptoms of liver cirrhosis include:
- Significant weight loss
- Loss of appetite
- Fatigue
- Weakness
- Itchy skin
- Yellow eyes and skin
- Nosebleeds
- Abdominal pain and swelling
- Swelling legs
- Confusion
- Enlargement of the breast in men

What Causes Fatty Liver?

Fatty liver occurs when the body is producing too much fat and it isn't being metabolized efficiently or fast enough. The excess fat is then stored in the liver where it can accumulate and cause the disease.

There are a variety of factors that can cause this fat build-up. As previously mentioned, drinking too much alcohol can cause AFLD, which is usually the initial stage of liver diseases that are associated with alcohol consumption.

But for people who drink alcohol in moderation or those that totally abstain from it and still develop NAFLD, the cause is less clear.

One or a few of these factors are considered to be potential causes:
- High blood sugar or diabetes
- Obesity
- Resistance to insulin
- High-fat levels in the blood, especially triglycerides

The following can also cause NAFLD but they're less common:
- Rapid weight loss
- Pregnancy
- Infections like hepatitis C
- Side effects due to certain medications which include tamoxifen, methotrexate, valproic acid, and amiodarone.
- Exposure to some toxins

Certain human genes have also been found to increase the risks of having NAFLD.

How is Fatty Liver Diagnosed?

Diagnosis of fatty liver include gathering the patient's medical history, conducting a physical exam, and doing one or more of the following tests:
- Blood test for elevated liver enzymes
- Imaging tests such MRI, CT scan, and ultrasound
- Liver biopsy

Fatty liver Treatment

There are currently no approved medications for the treatment of fatty liver. Fortunately, fatty liver is reversible in many cases and is easily accomplished by lifestyle changes like losing excess weight, avoiding or limiting alcohol, and making changes to the patient's diet.

Chapter 2 – Fatty Liver Diet

One of the most effective approaches to fatty liver is through losing excess body fat. Health experts agree that 70% of weight loss is due to diet.

Although there are no FDA approved drugs for the fatty liver yet, doctors agree that losing around 10% of the person's body weight is a good start, especially to patients who are obese.

NAFLD has been found most common for patients who live a sedentary lifestyle and those who consume mainly highly-processed foods.

Basic Components Of The Fatty liver Diet

A diet plan for people who have fatty liver should include the following:

- Lots of vegetables and fruits
- High-fiber foods like whole grains and legumes
- Reduced consumption of salt, sugar, refined carbohydrates, trans fat, and saturated fat
- No alcohol

Basically, the patient should undergo a reduced-calorie, low-fat diet to help in losing the excess weight.

Foods to Include in a Fatty liver Diet Plan

- **Greens**. In a study, broccoli has been found to be effective in helping prevent fat building in the livers of mice. Consuming more green vegetables like Brussels sprouts, spinach, and kale might also help with weight loss. There are a lot of vegetarian recipes that are full of flavor but low in calories.

- **Coffee**. Research has shown that those with fatty liver who also drink coffee are less susceptible to liver damage than those who don't. It's thought that the caffeine in this beverage reduces the levels of abnormal liver enzymes for those people that have high risks for liver diseases.

- **Fish**. Especially the fatty ones such as sardines, salmon, trout, and tuna, contain significant amounts of healthy omega-3 fatty acids. Omega-3 fatty acids have been found to help in improving fat levels in the liver and significantly reduce inflammation.

- **Tofu**. Soybeans have high protein content. Tofu is a soy product that has high protein content but a very low fat amount. A study made on rats by the University of Illinois showed that soy protein reduces liver fat buildup.

- **Walnuts**. These contain high amounts of omega-3 fatty acids which, as previously discussed, have shown to be beneficial in improving the liver function for patients diagnosed with fatty liver.

- **Oatmeal**. Carbohydrates consumed by patients with fatty liver should come from whole grains like oatmeal. Complex carbohydrates release a steady amount of energy and the fiber content satiates which is important in weight maintenance.

- **Low-fat dairy.** Whey protein might be able to help in protecting the liver from damage and this is important for those with fatty liver. Milk and other dairy products have high whey protein content but it's recommended those with reduced fat content.

- **Avocado**. It might be high in fat content but these are the healthy ones. Research suggests that healthy fats and certain chemicals found in avocado can slow down liver damage. Avocados are also fiber-rich which helps in weight control.

- **Olive oil**. It's one of the healthiest and more readily available oils in the market. Olive oil is rich in omega-3 fatty acids and is much healthier when used for food preparation compared to shortening, butter, or margarine. Research shows that it can lower the number of liver enzymes and also help control weight.

- **Sunflower seeds**. The vitamin E content of the nutty-tasting sunflower seeds can protect the liver from damage due to its anti-oxidant properties.

- **Green tea.** From aiding with sleep to lowering cholesterol, green tea has shown many medical and health benefits. Initial studies show that green tea helps by interfering with fat absorption. It might also help with improving liver function and reducing fat storage in the organ.

- **Garlic**. It doesn't just add a lot of flavor and aroma to food but garlic powder supplements are also showing potential in the reduction of excess body weight for people with fatty liver.

Foods to Avoid

The following foods should be avoided or the consumption limited for patients with fatty liver. These contribute to increased blood sugar levels and weight gain which should be avoided when treating the disease.

- Alcohol. It's not only the major cause for the disease but also for other organ diseases.
- Fried food. These are soaked in fat and generally high in calories.
- Added sugar. Sugary foods such as cookies, candies, fruit juices, and soda should be avoided. High levels of sugar in the blood can increase liver fat buildup.
- Pasta, rice, and bread. Especially the white ones because the flour used has been highly processed. These can raise blood sugar levels. Opt for brown rice and whole wheat bread and pasta.
- Salt. Salt is linked to water retention and also causes fat buildup and high blood pressure but it's an essential ingredient of most foods. Limit consumption to no more than 1.5 grams per day.

- Red meat. Avoid deli meats and beef because these have high saturated fat content.

Chapter 3 – Steps In Maintaining A Fatty liver Diet

Treating fatty liver with food is basically eating healthy. Here are some tips to consider for people with this condition

Eating Regular Meals

Eating regularly makes controlling appetite easier because it can reduce cravings and helps in planning healthy meals. Aim to have 3 meals per day.

Follow the Mediterranean Diet Pyramid

Fruits and vegetables, legumes, seeds, nuts, cereals, and wholegrain bread should take up most of the calories the patient consumes. Proteins should come from lean sources like fish, chicken breasts, and eggs. Low-fat dairy also provides additional protein, calcium, and other nutrients.

When the body gets enough nutrition coming from these food groups, craving for high sugar and high fat is greatly reduced.

Choose Healthier Drinks

Water is still the best beverage, especially for those people who are trying to lose weight. It contains zero calories and drinking a glass before a meal reduces food intake. Avoid drinks with too much sugar like juices, sports drinks, cordials, and sodas. Also, avoid alcohol as it can worsen fatty liver.

Reduce Portion Sizes

Replace that dinner plate with a salad plate. Studies show that the bigger the plate, the more food is consumed. Use smaller bowls and plates to reduce calorie intake.

Choose Healthier Alternatives

Eat more vegetables, fruits, legumes, and wholegrain, high-fiber cereals and bread. These satiate faster and longer but with fewer calories.

Here are examples of replacing food choices with better alternatives:
- Instead of a 1/3 bowl of muesli, eat a 2/3 bowl of oats
- Instead of a glass of fruit drink, eat 3 pieces of fruits
- Instead of 40 grams of chocolate, eat 2 slices multigrain bread

Both choices have the same calorie content but the latter is more filling than the former.

Plan Ahead

Planning meals ahead can help limit instances of impulse eating, the temptation of grabbing a takeaway, and other spur-of-the-moment food choices. Prepare a meal plan for the whole week and shop for the ingredients in the supermarket. Cooking meals and storing them in the refrigerator or freezer also helps a lot in controlling calorie intake.

Chapter 4 - Diet Plan And Sample Recipes for Fatty liver Patients

Sample Meal Plan

A typical meal plan for a patient with fatty liver might look like this:

Meal	Menu
Breakfast	- Hot oatmeal (8 oz.), mixed with almond butter (2 tsp.) and sliced banana (1 pc.) - Coffee with skim or low-fat milk (1 cup)
Lunch	- Salad greens with olive oil and balsamic vinegar dressing - Grilled chicken, 3 oz. - Baked small potato - Cooked carrots or broccoli, 1 cup - Apple, 1 pc. - Milk, 1 glass
Snack	- Raw veggies with 2 tbsp. of hummus or sliced apples with 1 tbsp. peanut butter
Dinner	- Mixed-bean salad, small - Grilled salmon, 3 oz. - Cooked broccoli, 1 cup - Whole-grain roll, 1 pc - Mixed berries, 1 cup - Milk, 1 glass

Another sample meal plan for a whole day:

Meal	Menu
Breakfast	- High-fiber cereal with low-fat milk or multigrain bread (2 slices) with tomato / baked beans / peanut butter / mushrooms / cottage cheese - Fruit, 1 pc. - Water
Morning Tea	- Fruit (1 pc) / Greek yogurt (100 – 200 g) / oatmeal biscuits (2 pcs.) / fruit bread (1 thin slice) / grainy crackers with tomato and cottage cheese (2 pcs.) / raw nuts (5 to 6 pcs.)
Lunch	- 1 wrap / 1 bread roll / multigrain bread (2 slices) - Green salad with low fat cheese / chicken / salmon / tuna - Water
Afternoon Tea	- Fruit (1 pc) / Greek yogurt (100 – 200 g) / oatmeal biscuits (2 pcs.) / fruit bread (1 thin slice) / grainy crackers with tomato and cottage cheese (2 pcs.) / raw nuts (5 to 6 pcs.)
Dinner	- 120 g lean chicken / eggs / chicken / legumes - Vegetables (zucchini / spinach / peas / cauliflower / carrots / cabbage / broccoli / beans - Whole wheat pasta (1 cup) / Brown rice (2/3cup) / sweet potato (1/2 cup) / medium potato (1 pc.) - Water

Just because you're going low-calorie does not mean you have to put up with bland food. There are ways to add flavor to any food without putting in too much salt or sugar. Here are some sample recipes that are low in calorie content but big in flavor.

Baked Salmon

Ingredients:
Lemons, 2 pcs, thinly sliced
Salmon fillet, (around 3 lbs.)
Kosher salt
Black pepper, freshly ground
Butter, melted, 6 tbsp.
Honey, 2 tbsp.
Garlic, minced, 3 cloves
Thyme leaves, chopped, 1 tsp.
Dried oregano, 1 tsp.
Fresh parsley, chopped, for garnish

Instructions:
1. Preheat the oven to 350 degrees. Use a foil to line a rimmed baking sheet. Grease it with cooking oil spray.
2. Lay the lemon slices on the center of the foil to form an even layer.
3. Season the salmon fillet on both sides with kosher salt and freshly ground black

pepper. Place fillet on top of the layer of lemon slices.

4. Whisk together oregano, thyme, garlic, honey, and butter in a small bowl. Pour this mixture over the salmon fillet and fold the foil up and around the salmon to form a packet.

5. Bake for 25 minutes or until the salmon is cooked through. Switch to broil and continue cooking for 2 more minutes.

6. Garnish with chopped fresh parsley and serve hot.

Grilled Chicken Breast

Ingredients:
Skinless, boneless, chicken breasts, 4 pcs.
Sugar, 1 tbsp.
Garlic powder, 1 tsp.
Italian seasoning, 2 tbsp.
Pepper, 1 tbsp.
Salt, 1 tbsp.
Lemon juice, 2 tbsp.
Worcestershire sauce, 3 tbsp.
Dijon mustard, 2 tbsp.
Cider vinegar, ¼ cup
Olive oil, 1/3 cup

Instructions:
1. Combine all of the ingredients in Ziploc bag or large bowl. Massage or toss until well combined.
2. Marinade the chicken breasts for at least 30 minutes. You can also refrigerate for up to 4 hours.
3. Preheat the grill to medium to medium-high heat.
4. Place marinated chicken breasts on the grill and cook for 7 to 8 minutes. Flip them over and cook for another 7 to 8 minutes. The internal temperature of the

chicken should be 165 degrees when checked with a meat thermometer.

5. Take the chicken off the grill and place in a serving plate. Let them rest for 3 to 5 minutes before slicing and serving.

Mixed Bean Salad

Ingredients:
Canned mixed bean salad, 400 g tin, drained and rinsed
Spring onions, 2 stalks, finely chopped
Celery, 2 sticks, thinly sliced
Tomato, large, 1 pc, deseeded then finely diced
Salt
Freshly ground black pepper
Dressing:
Olive oil, 3 tbsp
White wine vinegar, 1 tbsp
Sugar, 1 tsp
Dijon mustard, 2 tsp
Fresh tarragon, chopped, 1 tbsp
Fresh parsley, chopped, 1 tbsp

Instructions:
1. Put mixed beans, spring onions, celery, and tomato in a salad bowl. Add salt and pepper to taste. Mix well.
2. In a separate bowl, mix the ingredients for the dressing until well combined.
3. Pour the dressing on the salad and toss well together.

Chapter 5 – Lifestyle Changes

Treating fat liver disease and reversing the damage is all about lowering body weight. A 10 percent reduction in excess weight is enough to improve enzyme levels in the liver according to doctors.

Aside from the diet, another recommendation from doctors is for those with fatty liver to make a change in their lifestyles. Most patients diagnosed with NAFLD live a sedentary life with very little to no physical activity.

Here are some changes the patient should make to improve liver health.

Avoid Alcohol

This can't be reiterated enough. The liver goes through a lot of stress during alcohol consumption. Imagine that stress on an already diseased liver.

Lose Weight

But not rapidly. Losing 1 to 2 pounds per week should be the goal. Shedding off those extra pounds lower inflammation and prevents further injury to the liver.

Exercise

Aerobic has shown to be most effective in cutting fat levels in the liver. Walk, jog, or run regularly. Physical exercise also lowers inflammation. Exercise at least 3 times a week.

Manage Diabetes

For patients who are also suffering from diabetes, they should consult their doctor for proper management. The inability of the body to process sugar properly due to diabetes puts additional stress to the liver.

Lower Cholesterol Levels

Keep triglycerides and cholesterol levels down. This can be done through medication or eating a plant-based diet, and regular exercise.

Bonus Recipes

Green Smoothie

Ingredients

- 6 dandelion greens, chopped (about 1 cup)
- 4 kale leaves, stems removed and chopped (about 2 ½ cups)
- 1 Meyer or organic lemon, peeled and sliced into 1" chunks
- 1 small banana (optional) peeled and broken into 1" pieces
- 1 fuji apple, cut into 1" chunks
- 1 teaspoon grated ginger (optional)
- 2 cups Filtered water

Instructions

Place all ingredients, along with 2 cups water, into blender

Blend on high speed for 1-2 minutes until very smooth. Add more water as necessary.

Turkey sandwich

Ingredients

- 2 oz whole wheat pita bread
- 3 oz roasted turkey, sliced
- 2 slices tomato
- A few leaves of romaine lettuce
- 1 tsp mustard
- ½ C grapes

Detox Juice

Ingredients
1 beet, scrubbed
one handful of greens, washed (dandelion greens are also fine)
1 apple
1 cucumber, peeled
1 lemon, peeled

Instructions:

Juice all ingredients and stir

Lentil Soup

Ingredients:

1 tbsp (15 mL) vegetable oil
1 cup (250 mL) diced onion ½ cup (125 mL) diced carrot ½ cup (125 mL) diced celery 4 cups (1 L) vegetable or chicken broth 1 cup (250mL) dried red lentils, well rinsed ¼ tsp (1mL) dried thyme

Salt and freshly ground pepper ½ cup (125 mL) chopped fresh flat-leaf parsley 1.

Instructions:
In a large saucepan, heat oil over medium heat.

Sauté onion, carrot and celery until they are soft. This can be 5 minutes. Add broth, lentils and thyme. Then bring to a boil.

Reduce heat, cover and simmer for 20 minutes or until lentils are soft.

Remove from heat.

Transfer soup into a blender.

Purée on high speed until creamy.
Add up to 1 cup (250 mL) water if purée is too thick.

Season with salt and pepper and then return to saucepan to reheat, if necessary.

Ladle into bowls and garnish with parsley

Ragi Oat Crackers with a Cucumber Dip

For the ragi and oat crackers

1. Combine all the ingredients in a deep bowl and knead into a stiff dough using enough water.

2. Divide the dough into 2 equal portions

3. Roll out a portion into a 200 mm diameter circle without using any flour for rolling

4. Prick them all over using a fork and cut out into approximately small square pieces using a knife. You will get approximately 12 pieces

5. Repeat steps 3 and 4 to make 12 more pieces using another dough portion.

6. Arrange them on a greased baking tray and bake in a pre-heated oven at 180°c (360°f) for 25 to 30 minutes or till they turn crisp from both the sides, while turning them once after 12 minutes. Keep aside to cool slightly.

7. Store in an air-tight container and use as required.

Ingredients For The Ragi and Oat Crackers

1/2 cup ragi (nachni / red millet) flour

1/4 cup quick cooking rolled oats
1/2 cup whole wheat flour (gehun ka atta)
2 tsp olive oil
1/2 tsp green chili paste
1/2 tsp garlic (lehsun) paste salt to taste

To Be Mixed Into A Cucumber Dip
1/2 cup grated cucumber
1 cup hung low-fat curds (dahi) whisked
2 tbsp finely chopped mint leaves (phudina) leaves
2 tbsp finely chopped coriander (dhania)
1/4 tsp cumin seeds (jeera) powder
1/4 tsp garlic (lehsun) paste salt to taste
Method For the ragi and oat crackers

Combine all the ingredients in a deep bowl and knead into a stiff dough using enough water. Divide the dough into 2 equal portions.

Roll out a portion into a 200 mm. diameter circle without using any flour for rolling.

Prick them all over using a fork and cut out into approxately 2x2 pieces using a knife.

You will get approx. 12 pieces. Repeat steps 3 and 4 to make 12 more pieces using another dough portion.

Arrange them on a greased baking tray and bake in a pre-heated oven at 180°c (360°f) for 25 to 30 minutes or till they turn crisp from both the sides, while turning them once after 12 minutes.

Keep aside to cool slightly. Store in an air-tight container and use as required.

Conclusion

Fat liver disease is an easily preventable and treatable condition and it doesn't even require expensive medication or treatment methods. Basically, the patient just needs to eat a healthy, balanced diet and indulge in exercise to lower body weight and improve liver health.

Avoid consuming highly-processed foods which are usually loaded with salt, sugar, and fats. Instead opt for whole foods, especially fruits and vegetables. Cutting down or completely abstaining from alcohol is also required.

As the saying goes, prevention is always better than the cure and the same applies to fatty liver. Eating healthy and exercising regularly should be a conscious choice. These ensure the protection of not only the liver, but the whole body as well.

CPSIA information can be obtained
at www.ICGtesting.com
Printed in the USA
LVHW011144060221
678444LV00006B/702

9 781087 893112